The Pure Power *of*
MACA

Beverly Lynn Bennett

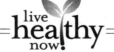

HEALTHY LIVING PUBLICATIONS
Summertown, Tennessee

Cover and interior design: Scattaregia Design

Healthy Living Publications,
a division of Book Publishing Company
PO Box 99
Summertown, TN 38483
888-260-8458
bookpubco.com

ISBN: 978-1-57067-336-8

Printed in the United States of America

20 19 18 17 16 15   1 2 3 4 5 6 7 8 9

Library of Congress Cataloging-in-Publication Data

Bennett, Beverly Lynn.
The pure power of maca / Beverly Lynn Bennett.
   pages cm
Includes index.
ISBN 978-1-57067-336-8 (pbk.) -- ISBN 978-1-57067-864-6 (e-book)
1. Materia medica, Vegetable. 2. Maca (Plant)--Health aspects. 3. Herbs--Therapeutic use. I. Title.
RS164.B425 2015
615.3'21--dc23
                2015025226

Printed on recycled paper

Book Publishing Company is a member of Green Press Initiative. We chose to print this title on paper with 100% post-consumer recycled content, processed without chlorine, which saved the following natural resources:

- 18 trees
- 563 pounds of solid waste
- 8,414 gallons of water
- 1,551 pounds of greenhouse gases
- 8 million BTUs of energy

For more information on Green Press Initiative, visit greenpressinitiative.org. Environmental impact estimates were made using the Environmental Defense Fund Paper Calculator. For more information, visit papercalculator.org.

Contents

Acknowledgments

I'd like to express my heartfelt appreciation to several people who helped make this book possible: Cynthia and Bob Holzapfel, my talented editor Jo Stepaniak, and the rest of the staff at Book Publishing Company, which publishes and produces so many fantastic vegan and vegetarian lifestyle books and cookbooks. I would also like to thank my family and friends for their love and support, especially my husband, Ray Sammartano, and my feline companion, Luna, for all their help during the recipe testing and writing of this book. And last but not least, to my fellow vegans, thank you for doing all that you can to spread the vegan message and for choosing to improve your lives and the lives of our fellow creatures who share this planet with us.

Introduction

Maca (*Lepidium meyenii*) is an herbaceous plant belonging to the brassica family, which includes broccoli, cabbage, collard greens, cauliflower, and kale. Unlike most of maca's relatives, the part of the plant that's consumed isn't the leaves or flowers but the starchy root tuber. The tuber resembles a radish in appearance, but its flavor is more like a slightly sweet potato. Maca grows in the high plateaus of the Andes Mountains in central Peru and Bolivia, where it has been cultivated for over three thousand years. In fact, maca and potatoes are the only two crops that actually thrive in the high altitudes and nutrient-rich volcanic soil of the Andes Mountains.

The Inca Indians of Peru consumed maca root on a daily basis, and it still remains an important dietary staple of the indigenous people of that area. The Incas often eat up to eight ounces of maca root a day, as it has the highest nutritional value of any food crop grown in the region. While fresh maca root can be eaten raw, in Peruvian culture, it's typically roasted in a fire pit, baked, or boiled to make it more digestible. After the initial cooking, it's sliced or mashed and used in porridges, soups, stews, puddings, or other savory or sweet dishes. The cooked and mashed maca root may also be blended with various liquids to make nourishing and tasty beverages, such as the popular fermented drink called *maca chicha*. For the Andean Indians, maca root is such a valuable commodity that they often used it to barter with communities living at lower elevations for other foods, such as beans, corn, fruits, leafy greens, other vegetables, quinoa, and rice.

Nutritional and Medicinal Benefits of Maca

The Incas discovered that maca has many medicinal as well as nutritional benefits. They observed that soon after eating maca, they felt more robust and energetic. According to legend, Incan warriors would consume large amounts of maca to help increase their strength and stamina before going into battle or embarking on long journeys. Within the Incan empire, maca was considered a powerful aphrodisiac that stimulates the libido of men and women and also increases their fertility. For these reasons, the Incas even started feeding maca to their animals.

Unknowingly, the Incas had stumbled upon a food source that is also a natural adaptogen. Adaptogens are an elite class of safe, nontoxic herbs used to improve the health of the adrenal system, which manages the body's hormonal response to stress. Adaptogens help balance and strengthen the body's ability to cope with anxiety and fight fatigue, but they do their work subtly and gently, without the jolts or crashes typical of drugs and chemicals.

There have been only a few double-blind randomized studies done with maca to date, and the majority of these studies have focused on maca's effects on the sexual function and libido of men and women. Therefore, most of the reported nutritional and medicinal benefits of maca are anecdotal, coming from athletes, consumers, nutritionists, and health care practitioners. Following are just a few of the reported benefits of taking maca:

- Heightens endurance and energy levels
- Boosts male libido
- Improves sexual function
- Decreases PMS and menopausal symptoms
- Supports overall brain health
- Enhances muscle-building capacity
- Reduces recovery time after exercise
- Increases mental focus and clarity
- Sharpens memory
- Elevates mood
- Eases depression
- Promotes a healthy immune system
- Regulates the endocrine glands

- Stimulates thyroid function
- Balances hormones
- Encourages hair growth
- Strengthens teeth and bones
- Heals acne
- Improves skin tone

Maca has been recommended by both conventional and alternative health care practitioners around the world since the 1980s. Some of the conditions they have prescribed maca for include anemia, chronic fatigue syndrome, HIV and AIDS, hormone imbalances, leukemia, osteoporosis, post-traumatic stress disorder, stomach cancer, other types of cancer, and tuberculosis. In traditional Chinese medicine, maca is considered a "warm" food because it strengthens, nourishes, and tonifies the body.

Maca is a rich source of several minerals, including calcium, iron, magnesium, and phosphorous. It also contains the trace minerals bismuth, copper, iodine, manganese, selenium, silica, and zinc, along with vitamins B_1, B_2, B_{12}, C, and E. Like other starchy vegetables, maca supplies carbohydrates, dietary fiber, essential fatty acids, lipids, plant sterols, and proteins, as well as trace to significant amounts of all twenty amino acids. In addition, maca contains four alkaloids proven in scientific studies to nourish the endocrine glands, including the reproductive systems of both men and women.

Maca is available in four forms: capsule, tablet, powder, and liquid extract (tincture). The capsules and tablets can be taken with water or juice, and the powder and extract can be added to foods or beverages. Because maca is a food, not a drug, herb, or supplement, most advocates contend that it's not possible to take too much of it. However, some people report increased heart rate and nervous energy when they consume a large dose, so it's wise to start with a conservative amount and increase the dosage slowly. When determining the quantity you should have, it's important to take into account your body weight, age, and general health. Large, young, active, healthy people can generally tolerate higher levels than small, elderly, sedentary, or ill individuals. Also bear in mind that maca affects different people differently, even those of the same weight, age, and levels of health and activity.

The most common recommended dose is 500 milligrams of maca taken one to three times per day. Because maca is an adaptogen, practitioners often suggest not using it continuously. Instead, they may recommend consuming it for one or two weeks and then taking a break from it for two or three days before resuming the cycle. An alternative approach is to consume it for three consecutive weeks and then take one week off. Note that recommended dosages of maca for therapeutic purposes are generally higher than for general health and immune support.

To date, there are no known toxic side effects from taking maca. However, as with most foods and supplements, people with certain health issues should heed a few cautions. Maca contains high levels of potassium, which may cause problems for individuals with renal insufficiencies. Maca also has high levels of natural iodine, which may cause thyroid problems in some individuals. While a small amount of iodine is necessary for thyroid function, too much can worsen the symptoms of thyroid disease. Like other members of the brassica family, maca is rich in glucosinolates, which can cause goiter in some individuals. People with thyroid disorders should check with their endocrinologist before consuming maca. Of course, as with any food or substance, it's possible to be allergic to maca. If you are prone to plant-based food allergies, you might want to consult your allergist before consuming maca.

High doses of maca should be used with caution, especially if you have high blood pressure, liver or kidney problems, or suffer from hormone-related cancers. If you experience any of these health problems, check with your doctor prior to using maca powder or supplements. Avoid taking maca if you are on hormone replacement therapy, taking contraceptives, or are pregnant or breastfeeding.

Varieties of Maca Root and Maca Powder

Maca is known by a variety of names, including ayak chichira, ayak willku, maca-maca, maino, maka, pepperweed, and Peruvian ginseng. Similar to radishes and turnips, the skin or peel of the maca root comes in a wide range of hues. The four most prevalent colors of the maca root are creamy yellow, light pink, deep purple, and gray-black. Because it is a vegetable, fresh maca root is highly perishable. To prolong its shelf life, manufacturers dry and grind it into a powder, a form that has rapidly gained worldwide popularity. The following list briefly describes each of the four types of maca powder available:

Cream maca powder. Creamy-yellow maca roots are the most commonly grown variety and make up the majority of the annual maca harvest. They're used to make cream maca powder, also known as yellow maca powder. This is the most widely available and least-expensive variety of maca powder.

Red maca powder. Light pink and dark purple maca roots are rarer. They're used to make red maca powder, which some people think has the mildest and sweetest taste. Studies have shown it to have the highest levels of phytonutrients and to be the best type of maca for hormone balancing. Red maca powder is highly recommended for women, as it helps with regulating the menstrual cycle. It's also purported to ease ovulation pain, improve libido, enhance fertility, and increase bone density and strength. In men, it's been shown to help support prostate health and prevent prostate cancer.

Black maca powder. The rarest maca roots are the ones that are light gray and dark gray-black. These are used for black maca powder, which, in studies, has proved to be the most effective in promoting memory, improving mental clarity and focus, facilitating muscle building, increasing bone density, and enhancing strength and endurance. Black maca powder is highly recommended for men, as it's been shown to heighten male libido and boost sperm count, volume, and motility.

Gelatinized maca powder. People who have sensitive stomachs or digestive problems may find that maca powder gives them gas, indigestion, or bloating. Gelatinized maca powder may be easier for them to digest than the other types. During the gelatinization process, the maca roots are boiled and pressurized to remove all of their starch content, which results in a more digestible and concentrated form of maca. However, some of maca's beneficial nutrients are altered and enzymes are destroyed from the high heat of this processing method. Despite the name, the gelatinization process does not involve the use of gelatin; therefore, gelatinized maca powder is suitable for use by vegans and vegetarians.

Surprisingly, maca's different skin pigments aren't apparent in the final product, as all of them, including gelatinized maca powder, are light tan in color. Most cream, red, and black maca powders are considered to be a raw-food product, because they're made from maca roots that have been sun-dried for several days prior to milling. Also, as the maca roots haven't been heated during processing, more of the beneficial enzymes, vitamins, and other nutrients are intact, which is why many consumers prefer to buy raw maca powders.

Cream, red, black, and gelatinized maca powders can all be found bulk-packaged for use in recipes, in addition to being sold in supplement form as capsules, tablets, or liquid extracts. They are all readily available through natural foods stores and online. I suggest trying various types of maca to determine which variety best suits your tastes and needs. Store maca powders or supplements in an airtight container away from direct sunlight, preferably in a cool, dark area with low humidity. Alternatively, to extend their shelf life, they can be stored in the refrigerator or freezer. Most companies that sell maca-based products state that they can be stored at room temperature for up to two years or in the refrigerator or freezer for up to two and a half years.

Using Maca Powder in Recipes

In this next section, you will learn more about how to use maca powder as a nutrient booster, flavor enhancer, binder, and flour in savory and sweet dishes. And in the recipe section that follows, I will share with you some of my favorite raw and cooked recipes, which run the gamut from beverages to desserts; of course, they all include the wondrous maca powder.

When you first sample maca powder, the flavor may seem a little unusual. Some people describe the taste as slightly sweet, others say it's mildly nutty or malty, and still others say it's reminiscent of caramel or butterscotch. I'm in the latter camp, and I've found that maca pairs beautifully with dishes that include vanilla, carob, or chocolate. Although all the recipes in this book contain maca, it's up to you whether to use the cream, red, black, or gelatinized powder; each of them will work equally well. If you opt to use cream, red, or black maca powder and find that you have excessive gas, indigestion, or bloating, try switching to gelatinized maca powder instead.

Keep in mind that no two people are the same, and maca will affect everyone a little differently. Some people will experience immediate health benefits, but for others it may take several weeks. If you're new to using maca powder in the kitchen, start slow. Incorporate small amounts of maca powder into dishes at first and work your way up to larger quantities. That way you can determine the quantity that appeals most to your taste buds, and you can also observe how your body reacts to maca. If you start to feel overly energized or jittery, simply cut back on the amount of maca powder you're using or take a brief break from it altogether.

When it comes to trying maca powder in recipes, a good starting point would be adding it to cold or hot beverages, such as fruit juices, herbal teas, and nondairy milks, shakes, and smoothies. Begin by adding one teaspoon of maca powder per serving and gradually work your way up to one tablespoon per serving. You can then move on to adding maca powder to your morning bowl of fruit, granola, oatmeal, or yogurt. Try mixing a few tablespoons into pancake or waffle batter to add a caramel flavor and energizing nutritional boost.

When you feel even more adventurous with your maca-enhanced culinary creations, start using maca powder as a binder or thickener in savory recipes, such as salad dressings, sauces, soups, stews, and veggie burgers. Or try it in sweet recipes, such as mousses, puddings, and raw energy bars. Maca powder can also be used to replace a portion of the flour in your favorite recipes for breads, cakes, cookies, crackers, muffins, and other baked goods.

In the pages ahead, you'll find a variety of recipes that I hope will inspire you to start adding maca powder to all your favorite breakfast, lunch, and dinner dishes, as well as to desserts, snacks, and treats. May this amazing superfood give you increased energy and vitality and greatly benefit your overall health and well-being.

Beverages

Superfood Smoothie

Yield: 2 servings

Start your day off right with this energizing smoothie. It features fruits, veggies, and a variety of popular superfoods that have anti-inflammatory and anticancer benefits. It's also packed with great flavor and abundant antioxidants, dietary fiber, essential fatty acids, vitamins, and minerals.

1½ cups leafy greens (such as kale, spinach, or a combination), lightly packed

1 cup coconut water

⅔ cup fresh or frozen blueberries, raspberries, or strawberries

⅔ cup fresh or frozen pineapple chunks

1 Hass avocado, halved

1 stalk celery, cut into 4 pieces

2 tablespoons goji berries

2 tablespoons hemp seeds

1 tablespoon chia seeds or flaxseeds

1 tablespoon maca powder

2 slices (¼ inch thick) fresh ginger (peeling optional)

½ teaspoon ground turmeric

Put all the ingredients in a blender in the order listed and process until smooth, stopping once to scrape down the blender jar. Serve immediately.

Variation: Replace the blueberries with 1 cup fresh or frozen pitted cherries.

Mocha-Maca Smoothie

Yield: 1 serving

Enjoy your morning cup of java a brand new way. This creamy smoothie beautifully marries the irresistible flavors of chocolate and coffee with the added boost of maca. If you're watching your caffeine intake, make it with decaf.

1 large banana, broken into 3 pieces

½ cup cold brewed coffee

½ cup ice cubes

⅓ cup plain, vanilla, or chocolate nondairy milk

1 tablespoon cacao powder or unsweetened cocoa powder

1 tablespoon maca powder

2 teaspoons agave nectar or unbleached cane sugar

½ teaspoon vanilla extract

⅛ teaspoon ground cinnamon

Put all the ingredients in a blender in the order listed and process until smooth, stopping once to scrape down the blender jar. Serve immediately.

Macadamia-Maca Malt

Yield: 1 serving

A malt is basically a milk shake enhanced with malted milk powder. Because maca powder has a slightly malty flavor, it's a natural malt alternative. Combined with macadamia nut milk and banana, it makes one heckuva classic soda-fountain drink.

1 cup water

⅓ cup macadamia nuts, soaked for 1 hour and drained

1 large banana, broken into 3 pieces

1 tablespoon maca powder

1 tablespoon agave nectar

4 ice cubes

1 teaspoon vanilla extract

Put the water and macadamia nuts in a blender and process for 1 minute. Scrape down the blender jar. Add the banana, maca powder, agave nectar, ice cubes, and vanilla extract and process until smooth, about 1 minute. Serve immediately.

Maca and Vanilla Milk Shake: Replace the banana with ½ cup of vanilla nondairy ice cream.

Nutty Nog

Yield: 4 servings

Eggnog is commonly served during the fall and winter holiday season, and this vegan version is just as rich and creamy as its egg- and dairy-laden counterpart. The caramel-like undertones of maca powder are complemented by a blend of spices, including turmeric, which gives this nog its familiar golden hue.

3 cups plain coconut milk beverage

⅓ cup raw cashew pieces or Brazil nuts, soaked for 1 hour and drained

¼ cup maple syrup or agave nectar

1 tablespoon maca powder

2 teaspoons vanilla extract

1 teaspoon ground cinnamon

½ teaspoon freshly grated nutmeg, plus more for garnish

¼ teaspoon ground ginger

¼ teaspoon ground cloves or allspice

¼ teaspoon ground turmeric

¼ cup Amaretto, bourbon, or rum (optional)

Put the milk and cashews in a blender and process for 1 minute. Scrape down the blender jar. Add the maple syrup, maca powder, vanilla extract, cinnamon, nutmeg, ginger, cloves, turmeric, and optional Amaretto and process until smooth, about 1 minute. Serve immediately or chill in the refrigerator. Garnish each serving with a sprinkle of additional nutmeg.

Pumpkin Nog: Add ⅔ cup of canned pumpkin purée.

Maca Chai Latte

Yield: 2 servings

Prepackaged chai is typically made with a combination of black tea and fragrant spices, such as cardamom, cinnamon, cloves, ginger, and nutmeg. Transform brewed chai into a creamy latte by blending it with maca powder, warm nondairy milk, and a touch of maple syrup.

1½ cups water

2 chai tea bags

1 cup plain coconut milk beverage or other nondairy milk

1½ tablespoons maple syrup or other sweetener

2 teaspoons maca powder

1 teaspoon vanilla extract

Put the water and tea bags in a small saucepan. Bring to a boil over high heat. Remove from the heat and let steep for 5 minutes. Remove and discard the tea bags.

While the tea is steeping, put the milk and maple syrup in a medium saucepan and heat over medium-high heat, stirring occasionally, until steaming hot and bubbles appear around the edges. Remove from the heat.

Transfer the milk mixture to a blender. Add the brewed tea, maca powder, and vanilla extract and process until frothy, stopping once to scrape down the blender jar. Alternatively, add the brewed tea, maca powder, and vanilla extract to the saucepan and use an immersion blender to process until frothy. Serve immediately.

Pumpkin-Maca Chai Latte: Add ¼ cup of canned pumpkin purée to the milk mixture as it heats.

Mexican Maca Hot Chocolate

Yield: 2 servings

In Mexico chocolate is commonly combined with spices to enrich its flavor. That tradition inspired this chocolaty beverage, which is enhanced with maca powder, cinnamon, and a little chili powder and cayenne to tingle your tongue and warm you up.

2 cups plain almond milk or other nondairy milk

2 tablespoons maca powder

¾ teaspoon ground cinnamon

½ teaspoon chili powder

Dash cayenne

1 cup vegan chocolate chips, or 2½ ounces Mexican chocolate, finely chopped

1 teaspoon vanilla extract

Dash sea salt

Put the milk, maca powder, cinnamon, chili powder, and cayenne in a medium saucepan and whisk until well combined. Bring to a boil over high heat. Remove from the heat and add the chocolate chips, vanilla extract, and salt. Whisk until the chocolate is completely melted. Serve immediately.

Variations: For a sweeter version, add 1 to 2 tablespoons of unbleached cane sugar, coconut sugar, or agave nectar. For a less spicy version, replace the chili powder and cayenne with ¼ teaspoon of ground nutmeg.

Breakfast and Brunch Ideas

Maca-Dusted Tropical Fruit Salad

Yield: 2 servings

This fruit salad will take your taste buds on a tropical vacation without ever leaving home. It's made with a blend of sweet and juicy fresh fruits and garnished with goji berries, macadamia nuts, and a dusting of maca-enhanced coconut sugar.

1 tablespoon coconut sugar

1½ teaspoons maca powder

1 large banana, thinly sliced

1 mango, peeled, pitted, and diced

⅔ cup pineapple chunks

1 kiwi, peeled, quartered lengthwise, and thinly sliced

¼ cup goji berries

¼ cup coarsely chopped macadamia nuts or other nuts

Put the coconut sugar and maca powder in a small bowl and stir until well combined.

Put the banana, mango, pineapple, and kiwi in a medium bowl and toss gently. Sprinkle the goji berries, macadamia nuts, and maca mixture over the top. Serve immediately.

Variation: Replace the goji berries with ¼ cup of pomegranate seeds.

Berry and Cream Breakfast Parfaits

Yield: 2 servings

A luscious cream made with chia and hemp seeds is layered with fresh berries to create healthy, eye-popping parfaits. Serve this colorful treat for breakfast or dessert.

  1 cup water

  ¼ cup chia seeds

  ¼ cup hemp seeds

  4 pitted soft dates, soaked for 30 minutes and drained

  2 teaspoons maca powder

  1 teaspoon vanilla extract

  1 cup sliced strawberries

  ½ cup blueberries

  ½ cup raspberries or blackberries

To make the cream, put the water, chia seeds, hemp seeds, dates, maca powder, and vanilla extract in a blender and process until smooth, stopping once to scrape down the blender jar. Transfer to a small bowl and set aside for 15 minutes. Just before using, whisk the mixture to break up any clumps of chia seeds.

To assemble the parfaits, have ready two tall glasses. In each glass, layer one-quarter of the cream, ¼ cup of the strawberries, 2 tablespoons of the blueberries, and 2 tablespoons of the raspberries. Repeat the layers with the remaining cream and berries. Serve immediately.

Variation: Replace the strawberries, blueberries, and blackberries with chopped fruit, such as bananas, cherries, peaches, persimmons, plums, or kiwis.

Stewed Caramel Apples

Yield: 3 cups

Fill your house with the sweet-smelling aroma of apple pie but with minimal effort. This naturally sweetened treat can be served warm or cold as a side dish or as a topping for hot cereal, toast, pancakes, waffles, nondairy ice cream, or cake.

    4 cups peeled and sliced apples
    1 cup apple juice
    6 pitted soft dates, soaked for 30 minutes, drained, and
       coarsely chopped
    2 tablespoons maca powder
    1 teaspoon ground cinnamon
    1 teaspoon vanilla extract

Put the apples, apple juice, dates, maca powder, and cinnamon in a medium saucepan and cook over medium heat, stirring occasionally, until the apples are tender, 8 to 10 minutes. Stir in the vanilla extract and remove from the heat. Serve warm or cold.

Variation: Replace the dates with ⅓ cup of raisins or dried cranberries.

Stewed Caramel Pears: Replace the apples with 4 cups of peeled and sliced pears.

Fruit-n-Nut Granola

Yield: 8 cups

Enjoy this crunchy and slightly sweet blend of oats, shredded coconut, nuts, seeds, and dried fruit as a cold breakfast cereal topped with nondairy milk or yogurt. This granola also works great as a topping for fresh fruit salad, nondairy ice cream, and sorbet.

4 cups old-fashioned rolled oats

1 cup coarsely chopped nuts (such as almonds, pecans, or walnuts)

½ cup unsweetened shredded dried coconut

½ cup raw sunflower seeds

¼ cup hemp seeds

¾ cup apple juice

½ cup maple syrup or agave nectar

¼ cup maca powder

3 tablespoons sunflower or safflower oil

1 tablespoon ground cinnamon

1 tablespoon vanilla extract

1 cup dried fruit (such as raisins, cranberries, chopped apricots, or chopped dates)

Preheat the oven to 350 degrees. Line a baking sheet with parchment paper or a silicone baking mat.

Put the oats, nuts, coconut, sunflower seeds, and hemp seeds in a large bowl and stir to combine. Put the apple juice, maple syrup, maca powder, oil, cinnamon, and vanilla extract in a small bowl or measuring cup and whisk until well combined. Pour the apple juice mixture over the oat mixture and stir until well combined. Transfer to the lined baking sheet and spread into a single layer.

Bake for 20 minutes. Remove from the oven, stir, and spread into a single layer again. Bake for 20 to 25 minutes longer, until golden brown and dry. Remove from the oven, sprinkle the dried fruit over the top, and stir until evenly distributed. Let cool completely. Stored in a sealed container at room temperature, Fruit-n-Nut Granola will keep for 1 month.

Chunky Monkey Maca Bread

Yield: 1 loaf, 8 servings

This scrumptious quick bread recipe combines three popular ingredients: bananas, chocolate, and walnuts. Indulge in a generous slice or two for breakfast, or serve it for dessert topped with nondairy yogurt or your favorite nondairy ice cream.

⅔ cup plain almond milk or other nondairy milk

1 tablespoon cider vinegar

2 cups whole wheat pastry flour

⅔ cup coconut sugar

3 tablespoons maca powder

2 teaspoons baking soda

1 teaspoon ground cinnamon

¼ teaspoon sea salt

2 large, very ripe bananas, coarsely mashed

1½ teaspoons vanilla extract

½ cup vegan chocolate chips or carob chips

½ cup coarsely chopped walnuts

Preheat the oven to 350 degrees F. Lightly oil an 8 x 4 x 2½-inch loaf pan or mist it with cooking spray.

Put the milk and vinegar in a small bowl and stir until well combined. Set aside for 5 minutes to thicken.

Put the flour, coconut sugar, maca powder, baking soda, cinnamon, and salt in a large bowl and whisk until well combined. Add the milk mixture, bananas, and vanilla extract and whisk until well combined. Gently stir in the chocolate chips and walnuts. Pour into the prepared loaf pan.

Bake for 45 to 55 minutes, or until a toothpick inserted in the center comes out clean. Let the bread cool slightly before removing it from the pan and slicing. Stored in a sealed container at room temperature, Chunky Monkey Maca Bread will keep for 3 days.

Gluten-Free Chunky Monkey Maca Bread: Replace the whole wheat pastry flour with 2 cups of gluten-free all-purpose flour and ¾ teaspoon xanthan gum.

Maca-Maple Pancakes

Yield: 8 pancakes

Maple syrup, maca powder, cinnamon, and vanilla extract add the perfect touch of sweetness and spiciness to these fluffy pancakes. Serve them with your choice of toppings, such as vegan butter, jam, maple or fruit-based syrup, or fresh fruit or berries.

1½ cups whole wheat pastry flour or unbleached flour

2 tablespoons maca powder

1 tablespoon aluminum-free baking powder

1½ teaspoons ground cinnamon

½ teaspoon sea salt

1½ cups plain soy milk or other nondairy milk

1½ tablespoons maple syrup

1 tablespoon safflower oil or other oil

1½ teaspoons vanilla extract

1 teaspoon cider vinegar

Put the flour, maca powder, baking powder, cinnamon, and salt in a large bowl and whisk until well combined. Add the milk, maple syrup, oil, vanilla extract, and vinegar and whisk until well combined. Set aside for 5 minutes.

Lightly oil a large cast iron or nonstick skillet or griddle or mist it with cooking spray. Heat over medium heat. When the skillet is hot, pour the batter into it using a ⅓ cup of batter for each pancake. You will need to cook the pancakes in several batches depending on the size of the skillet. Cook until the edges of the pancakes are slightly dry and bubbles appear on the top, 2 to 3 minutes. Flip the pancakes over with a spatula and cook until golden brown on the other side, 2 to 3 minutes. Lightly oil the skillet again and repeat with the remaining batter. Serve hot.

Variation: Add coarsely chopped nuts or seeds, chopped or sliced fresh fruit, fresh or frozen berries, or vegan chocolate or carob chips.

Peruvian-Style Potato Skillet

Yield: 6 cups, 4 servings

Thousands of varieties of potatoes are grown in Peru. In this Peruvian-inspired recipe, the visually striking purple potato is paired with corn, peppers, chiles, and spices, which are all commonly used in the region. Serve this as a side dish for breakfast or dinner.

1½ pounds purple potatoes, scrubbed and cubed

1½ tablespoons olive oil or other oil

1 large zucchini, quartered lengthwise and sliced

1 cup diced red bell pepper

1 cup diced yellow or orange bell pepper

1 cup fresh or frozen corn kernels

1 jalapeño chile, seeded and finely diced

1 teaspoon chili powder

1 teaspoon ground coriander

1 teaspoon ground cumin

⅓ cup chopped fresh cilantro, lightly packed

2 tablespoons maca powder

1 tablespoon nutritional yeast flakes

Sea salt

Freshly ground black pepper

Hot pepper sauce

Put the potatoes and oil in a large cast iron or nonstick skillet and cook over medium-high heat, stirring occasionally, for 10 minutes. Add the zucchini, red bell pepper, yellow bell pepper, corn, and chile and cook, stirring occasionally, until the vegetables are tender, 5 to 7 minutes.

Add the chili powder, coriander, and cumin and cook, stirring occasionally, for 1 minute. Add the cilantro, maca powder, and nutritional yeast and stir until well combined. Remove from the heat. Season with salt, pepper, and hot pepper sauce to taste. Serve hot.

Snacks, Sides, and Main Dishes

Savory Flax and Sesame Crackers

Yield: 54 crackers

Almond meal, chickpea flour, maca powder, dried herbs, and flax and sesame seeds work in unison to create the savory flavor of these gluten-free crackers. Munch them by the handful or serve them as an accompaniment to your favorite vegan cheeses, dips, and spreads.

¾ cup almond meal

¾ cup chickpea flour

⅓ cup flaxseeds

⅓ cup sesame seeds

3 tablespoons maca powder

1½ tablespoons nutritional yeast flakes

1 tablespoon Italian seasoning

⅓ cup water

1½ tablespoons toasted sesame oil or other oil

1 tablespoon reduced-sodium tamari

Preheat the oven to 375 degrees F.

Put the almond meal, chickpea flour, flaxseeds, sesame seeds, maca powder, nutritional yeast, and Italian seasoning in a medium bowl and stir until well combined. Add the water, oil, and tamari and stir until the mixture forms a soft, slightly sticky dough.

Put the dough between two large pieces of parchment paper or two silicone baking mats. Using a rolling pin, roll the dough into an 18 x 12-inch rectangle, about ⅛ inch thick. Remove and discard the top sheet of parchment paper. Score the dough into 2-inch squares with a knife or pizza cutter; do not separate the squares.

Transfer the parchment paper to a baking sheet. Bake for 10 to 12 minutes, until the crackers are dry and lightly browned. Let cool completely before gently separating the scored crackers. Stored in a sealed container at room temperature, Savory Flax and Sesame Crackers will keep for 5 days.

Garden Guaca-Maca-Mole

Yield: 2 cups, 4 servings

In this guacamole, maca powder and avocado work as tag-team nutrition boosters while also aiding the body's absorption of fat-soluble nutrients, specifically the carotenoids beta-carotene, lutein, and lycopene, which are found in tomatoes and bell peppers. Serve this dip as a snack or appetizer with tortilla chips and salsa, or as a condiment.

2 Hass avocados, halved

Zest and juice of 1 lime

1 tablespoon minced garlic

¼ cup finely diced red onion

¼ cup finely diced orange or yellow bell pepper

¼ cup finely diced tomato

¼ cup chopped fresh cilantro, lightly packed

2 tablespoons maca powder

Sea salt

Freshly ground black pepper

Put the avocados, lime zest and juice, and garlic in a medium bowl and mash with a fork until very smooth. Add the onion, bell pepper, tomato, cilantro, and maca powder and stir until well combined. Season with salt and pepper to taste.

Creamy Mushroom and Maca Soup

Yield: 8 cups, 6 servings

Looking to boost your libido? Then give this recipe a try, as it features many foods that are considered to be aphrodisiacs, including maca, mushrooms, onions, celery, and garlic. The final addition of coconut milk creamer and optional white wine heightens the aroma of this creamy, delicately flavored soup.

> 1 cup diced yellow onion
> 1 cup diced celery
> 1½ tablespoons olive oil
> 12 ounces button or crimini mushrooms, halved and thinly sliced
> 1½ tablespoons minced garlic
> 6 tablespoons unbleached flour or other flour
> 2½ tablespoons maca powder
> 4 cups no-salt-added vegetable broth
> ⅓ cup chopped fresh parsley, lightly packed
> 2 tablespoons chopped fresh thyme, or 2 teaspoons dried
> 1 cup plain coconut milk creamer or nondairy milk
> 2 tablespoons white wine or sherry (optional)
> 1 tablespoon nutritional yeast flakes
> Sea salt
> Freshly ground black pepper

Put the onion, celery, and oil in a large soup pot and cook over medium-high heat, stirring occasionally, until softened, about 3 minutes. Add the mushrooms and garlic and cook, stirring occasionally, for 5 minutes.

Sprinkle the flour and maca powder over the vegetable mixture and cook, stirring occasionally, for 2 minutes. Slowly stir in the vegetable broth, parsley, and thyme. Increase the heat to high and bring to a boil. Decrease the heat to low, cover, and simmer until the mushrooms are tender, about 20 minutes.

Stir in the creamer, optional wine, and nutritional yeast and cook, stirring frequently, for 2 minutes longer. Season with salt and pepper to taste.

Creamy Mushroom, Barley, and Maca Soup: When adding the vegetable broth, add ⅓ cup of hulled or pearled barley, rinsed. Simmer the soup until the barley is tender, about 30 minutes. Continue with the recipe as directed.

Almond Butter Sauce

Yield: 1½ cups

Lime juice and vinegar add a pleasingly tangy complement to the malty maca powder and zippy fresh ginger in this creamy sauce. This versatile condiment can be used as a dressing for salads and slaws or as a sauce for cooked noodles and steamed or stir-fried vegetables.

½ cup water

½ cup almond butter

⅓ cup reduced-sodium tamari

Zest and juice of 2 limes

2 tablespoons maca powder

2 tablespoons brown rice vinegar

2 tablespoons toasted sesame oil

1½ tablespoons peeled and grated fresh ginger

¼ teaspoon freshly ground black pepper

Put all the ingredients in a medium bowl and whisk until well combined. Use immediately or refrigerate for 15 minutes before serving to thicken the sauce slightly. Stored in a sealed container in the refrigerator, Almond Butter Sauce will keep for 7 days.

Variation: Replace the almond butter with another nut or seed butter, such as cashew, hazelnut, peanut, or sunflower butter.

Crunchy Veggie Salad with Almond Butter Dressing

Yield: 8 cups, 4 servings

This colorful salad features a blend of crisp and crunchy fresh vegetables tossed with Almond Butter Sauce. Leftovers make a great filling for sandwiches or wraps.

2½ cups small broccoli florets

2 cups shredded savoy or green cabbage

2 cups shredded red cabbage

2 carrots, halved lengthwise and thinly sliced on a diagonal

2 stalks celery, thinly sliced on a diagonal

¾ cup diced red bell pepper

½ cup snow peas, cut in half on a diagonal

⅔ cup Almond Butter Sauce (page 31)

2 tablespoons water

Put the broccoli, savoy cabbage, red cabbage, carrots, celery, bell pepper, and snow peas in a large bowl and toss gently to combine.

Put the Almond Butter Sauce and water in a small bowl and whisk until well combined. Pour over the vegetable mixture and toss gently until the vegetables are evenly coated. Serve immediately.

Variation: For a heartier salad, add cubed baked or fried tofu or cooked noodles or grains.

Maca-Roasted Rutabagas and Turnips

Yield: 6 cups, 6 servings

Because maca is a root vegetable, it seems only fitting to pair it with other root vegetables, such as rutabagas and turnips. In this recipe these tasty roots are lightly seasoned and dusted with maca powder, then oven-roasted to perfection to bring out their natural sweetness.

2 pounds rutabagas, peeled and cut into 2-inch cubes

2 pounds turnips, peeled and cut into 2-inch cubes

2 tablespoons olive oil or toasted sesame oil

2 tablespoons maca powder

1 tablespoon garlic powder

1 teaspoon sea salt

½ teaspoon freshly ground black pepper

Preheat the oven to 400 degrees F. Line a baking sheet with parchment paper or a silicone baking mat.

Arrange the rutabagas and turnips in a single layer on the lined baking sheet. Drizzle the oil evenly over the vegetables. Sprinkle the maca powder, garlic powder, salt, and pepper over the top. Using your hands, toss until evenly coated, then spread into a single layer.

Bake for 25 minutes. Remove from the oven, stir with a spatula, and spread into a single layer. Bake for 20 to 25 minutes longer, until the vegetables are tender and lightly browned around the edges.

Maca-Roasted Carrots and Parsnips: Replace the rutabagas and turnips with 2 pounds each of carrots and parsnips, peeled and cut into 2-inch cubes.

Incan-Style Quinoa and Bean Patties

Yield: 12 patties

These savory, gluten-free patties are made with a combination of red beans, tricolor quinoa, a colorful blend of vegetables, cornmeal, maca powder, and an ample amount of seasonings. Serve them as an entrée or on buns, plain or with your favorite condiments and toppings.

¼ cup water

1 tablespoon chia seeds

1 can (15 ounces) red, black, kidney, or pinto beans, drained and rinsed

1½ cups cooked tricolor quinoa or other quinoa, cooled

1 cup peeled and finely diced sweet potato

½ cup finely diced red bell pepper

½ cup fresh or frozen corn kernels

½ cup thinly sliced green onions

½ cup chopped fresh cilantro, lightly packed

1 jalapeño chile, seeded and finely diced

Zest and juice of 1 lime

2 tablespoons minced garlic

1 tablespoon chili powder or ancho chile powder

1 tablespoon ground cumin

1 teaspoon sea salt

½ teaspoon freshly ground black pepper

¼ cup cornmeal

¼ cup maca powder

Put the water and chia seeds in a large bowl and whisk to combine. Set aside for 10 minutes to thicken. Add ¾ cup of the beans and coarsely mash with a fork.

Add the remaining beans, quinoa, sweet potato, bell pepper, corn, green onions, cilantro, chile, lime zest and juice, garlic, chili powder, cumin, salt, and pepper and stir until well combined. Add the cornmeal and maca powder and stir until well combined.

Line a large baking sheet with parchment paper. Using a ¼-cup measuring cup and wet hands, portion the mixture into 12 patties, putting them on the lined baking sheet as they are made. Moisten your hands with water between shaping and flattening each patty. Chill the patties in the refrigerator for 30 minutes.

Preheat the oven to 400 degrees F. Bake the patties on the lined baking sheet for 15 minutes. Flip them over with a spatula and bake for 10 to 15 minutes longer, until lightly browned on both sides.

Pumpkin Maca-roni and Cheese

Yield: 6 servings

Using canned pumpkin purée is a great way to enhance the nutritional value of the cheesy sauce in this recipe as well as give it a natural orange hue. This may become your go-to recipe when you're in need of some quick and simple comfort food.

12 ounces macaroni or other small pasta

⅓ cup nutritional yeast flakes

2 tablespoons maca powder

1 tablespoon tapioca starch

1 teaspoon sea salt

½ teaspoon paprika

½ teaspoon garlic powder

½ teaspoon onion powder

¼ teaspoon freshly ground black pepper

1½ cups unsweetened plain nondairy milk

¾ cup canned pumpkin purée

Cook the macaroni in boiling water according to the package directions. Drain in a colander.

While the macaroni is cooking, make the sauce. Put the nutritional yeast, maca powder, tapioca starch, salt, paprika, garlic powder, onion powder, and pepper in a large saucepan and whisk to combine. Add the milk and whisk until well combined. Cook over medium heat, whisking occasionally, until the sauce thickens, 3 to 5 minutes.

Whisk in the pumpkin purée and remove from the heat. Add the cooked macaroni and stir until well combined. Heat over medium-low heat, stirring frequently, until hot.

Variation: Replace the pumpkin purée with ¾ cup of canned butternut squash or sweet potato purée.

Extra-Cheesy Pumpkin Maca-roni: Add 1 cup of shredded vegan Cheddar cheese.

Sweets and Treats

Salted Caramel Nut Bars

Yield: 12 bars

The caramel flavor of these bars is achieved by blending almonds, dates, maca powder, and vanilla extract. The shaped bars are garnished with a fine dusting of Himalayan pink salt to heighten the flavor of these totally raw treats.

2 cups raw whole almonds

1 cup pitted soft dates, soaked for 30 minutes and drained

1 tablespoon maca powder

1 tablespoon vanilla extract

Himalayan pink salt

Put the almonds in a food processor and pulse until coarsely chopped. Remove half the almonds and put them in a medium bowl.

Add the dates, maca powder, and vanilla extract to the remaining almonds in the food processor and process until finely ground, 1 to 2 minutes. Scrape down the container and continue processing until the mixture holds together when gently squeezed between your fingers, about 1 minute. Using your hands, work the date mixture into the reserved chopped almonds until well combined.

Put a piece of parchment paper on a large cutting board. Divide the mixture in half and transfer each half to the cutting board. Using your hands, pat each half into a 9 x 4-inch rectangle. Refrigerate until firm, about 1 hour.

When firm, cut each rectangle into 6 bars, each about 4 x 1½ inches. Lightly sprinkle a little Himalayan pink salt over each bar. Stored in a sealed container in the refrigerator, Salted Caramel Nut Bars will keep for 7 days.

Chocolate or Carob Salted Caramel Nut Bars: Melt ⅓ cup of vegan chocolate chips or carob chips in the microwave or a double boiler. Spread the melted chips over the cut bars, then lightly sprinkle the tops with a little Himalayan pink salt.

Bliss Balls

Yield: 16 balls

These coconut-covered confections are made with a wholesome blend of dried fruits, nuts, and seeds. They're spiked with the zest and juice of a satsuma orange (a type of mandarin), invigorating ground ginger, and maca powder. Enjoy these nutritious morsels as an afternoon snack or a sweet treat. They'll give you an extra boost after exercising.

1¼ cups raisins

1 cup dried apricots

½ cup raw cashew pieces or other nuts

½ cup raw sunflower seeds

¼ cup hemp seeds

1½ tablespoons maca powder

½ teaspoon ground ginger

1 cup unsweetened shredded dried coconut

Zest and juice of 1 satsuma or other mandarin orange

Put the raisins, apricots, cashews, sunflower seeds, hemp seeds, maca powder, and ginger in a food processor and process until finely ground, 1 to 2 minutes. Add ⅔ cup of the coconut and the satsuma zest and juice and process until the mixture comes together to form a ball, about 1 minute.

Put the remaining ⅓ cup of coconut in a small bowl. Using wet hands, form the apricot mixture into 1-inch balls. Roll each ball in the coconut until evenly coated on all sides. Stored in a sealed container, Bliss Balls will keep for 7 days in the refrigerator or 3 months in the freezer.

Maca-roons

Yield: 20 cookies

People who follow a gluten-free and egg-free diet will adore the luscious, rich flavor of these cookies. They're made with a combination of coconut, coconut milk, and almond meal, and are lightly sweetened with agave nectar. A liberal amount of maca powder adds an extra dimension of flavor to these moist and chewy treats.

2½ cups unsweetened shredded dried coconut

⅔ cup almond meal

¼ cup maca powder

¼ teaspoon sea salt

½ cup lite coconut milk

6 tablespoons agave nectar

1½ teaspoons vanilla extract

Preheat the oven to 350 degrees F. Line a baking sheet with parchment paper or a silicone baking mat.

Put the coconut, almond meal, maca powder, and salt in a medium bowl and stir with a fork to combine. Add the coconut milk, agave nectar, and vanilla extract and stir until well combined.

Drop the dough onto the lined baking sheet using 2 tablespoons, very firmly packed, for each cookie. Space the cookies 2 inches apart.

Bake for 18 to 20 minutes, until golden brown on the bottom and around the edges. Let the cookies cool completely on the baking sheet. Stored in a loosely covered container at room temperature, Maca-roons will keep for 5 days.

Chocolate or Carob Chip Maca-roons: Add ⅔ cup of vegan chocolate chips or carob chips.

Power-Up-the-Trail Cookies

Yield: 18 cookies

Use your favorite trail mix or your own combination of dried fruits, nuts, and seeds to create these gluten-free cookies. They'll keep you well fueled and energized for hours.

> ½ cup tahini or other seed or nut butter
>
> ½ cup maple syrup or agave nectar
>
> 3 tablespoons maca powder
>
> 1 tablespoon vanilla extract
>
> 1½ cups old-fashioned rolled oats
>
> 1 cup trail mix or a combination of dried fruits, nuts, and seeds
>
> ¼ cup unsweetened shredded dried coconut

Preheat the oven to 350 degrees. Line two baking sheets with parchment paper or silicone baking mats.

Put the tahini, maple syrup, maca powder, and vanilla extract in a large bowl and stir until well combined. Add the oats, trail mix, and coconut and stir until well combined.

Drop the dough onto the lined baking sheets using 2 tablespoons for each cookie, spacing them 2 inches apart. Using wet fingers, flatten each cookie slightly.

Bake for 15 minutes, until golden brown on the bottom and around the edges. Let cool for 2 minutes on the baking sheets before transferring to a rack to cool completely. Stored in an airtight container at room temperature, Power-Up-the-Trail Cookies will keep for 5 days.

Raw Chocolates with Maca

Yield: 12 to 20 pieces

Get ready to feel like a real chocolatier, as it's quite easy to make your own homemade raw chocolates. These rich, dark morsels are made with a blend of cocoa butter, cacao powder, and maca powder and are sweetened with agave nectar. Food-grade cocoa butter is readily available online, at natural foods stores, or any store that sells confectionery or baking supplies.

    3 ounces (6 tablespoons) cocoa butter or coconut oil

    ¼ cup cacao powder or unsweetened cocoa powder

    1½ tablespoons maca powder

    1½ tablespoons agave nectar

    1 teaspoon vanilla extract

    Dash Himalayan pink salt or sea salt

Fill one-quarter of the lower portion of a double boiler with water and put over low heat. Put the cocoa butter in the top part of the double boiler and gently heat until just melted, 3 to 5 minutes.

Remove the the top part of the double boiler. Add the cacao powder, maca powder, agave nectar, vanilla extract, and salt to the melted cocoa butter and whisk until well combined.

Evenly portion the chocolate mixture into candy molds or an ice-cube tray. Put in the refrigerator or freezer until the chocolate is set, about 1 hour. Stored in a sealed container in the refrigerator, Raw Chocolates with Maca will keep for 1 month.

Tip: If you don't have a double boiler, you can improvise one by filling a small saucepan with 1 inch of water. Put a small, shallow bowl on top of the saucepan, making sure the water doesn't touch the bottom of the bowl.

Chocolate-Maca Mousse

Yield: 1 serving

Made with just six ingredients, this simple avocado-based mousse is ideal for chocoholics who want to enjoy their chocolate without it adding to their waistlines. Savor this single-serving treat plain or topped with fresh berries, chopped nuts, or shredded coconut.

1 Hass avocado

2 tablespoons cacao powder or unsweetened cocoa powder

2 tablespoons agave nectar or maple syrup

1 teaspoon maca powder

½ teaspoon vanilla extract

Dash Himalayan pink salt or sea salt

Put the avocado, cacao powder, agave nectar, maca powder, vanilla extract, and salt in a food processor and process until completely smooth, 1 to 2 minutes. Scrape down the container and process for 30 seconds longer.

Transfer to a glass bowl. Serve immediately or chill in the refrigerator for 30 minutes before serving.

Carob-Maca Mousse: Replace the cacao powder with 2 tablespoons of unsweetened carob powder.

Easy Banana and Maca Ice Cream

Yield: 1 serving

There's no need for an ice-cream maker to create spectacular frozen desserts. Simply blend a frozen banana in a food processor and you'll have dairy-free soft-serve ice cream in minutes. It's sweet, creamy, and 100 percent natural—the ideal treat for every sweet tooth.

1 large, very ripe banana, frozen

1½ teaspoons maca powder

½ teaspoon vanilla extract

1 to 2 teaspoons water or nondairy milk

Break the banana into 3 pieces. Put the banana, maca powder, and vanilla extract in a food processor and process for 1 minute. Scrape down the container. If the mixture is too thick, add 1 teaspoon of water at a time and process again until the desired consistency is achieved, 30 to 60 seconds. Serve immediately.

Cacao Chip-Maca Ice Cream: Add 2 tablespoons of cacao nibs to the finished ice cream and stir gently to combine.

Peanut Butter, Banana, and Maca Ice Cream: Add 1 tablespoon of peanut butter and process with the banana mixture.

Strawberry, Banana, and Maca Ice Cream: Use only ½ of a banana and add ½ cup of fresh or frozen strawberries.

Maca Spice Cake

Yield: 1 cake, 8 servings

The slight butterscotch flavor of maca powder is elevated by combining it with applesauce, cinnamon, ginger, and allspice in this fat-free spice cake. Serve it plain or topped with nondairy yogurt, your favorite frosting, or Easy Banana and Maca Ice Cream (page 43).

1½ cups whole wheat pastry flour or unbleached flour
⅔ cup unbleached cane sugar
¼ cup maca powder
1½ teaspoons baking soda
1 teaspoon ground cinnamon
½ teaspoon ground ginger
½ teaspoon ground allspice
¼ teaspoon sea salt
1 cup applesauce
½ cup apple juice or water
1½ teaspoons vanilla extract
1 tablespoon cider vinegar

Preheat the oven to 350 degrees F. Lightly oil an 8-inch round or square baking pan or mist it with cooking spray.

Put the flour, sugar, maca powder, baking soda, cinnamon, ginger, allspice, and salt in a large bowl and whisk to combine. Add the applesauce, apple juice, and vanilla extract and whisk until completely smooth. Add the vinegar and whisk until well combined. Pour into the prepared baking pan.

Bake for 25 to 30 minutes, or until a toothpick inserted in the center comes out clean. Serve warm or at room temperature. Stored at room temperature in a sealed container or tightly covered with plastic wrap, Maca Spice Cake will keep for 3 days.

Sweet Potato and Maca Spice Cake: Replace the applesauce with 1 cup of canned sweet potato purée.

Recipe Index

About the Author

Beverly Lynn Bennett is a vegan chef and baker who is passionate about creating easy, delicious, and healthy vegan recipes. Beverly is the author of several books, including *Vegan Bites: Recipes for Singles, Chia: Using the Ancient Superfood, Kale: The Nutritional Powerhouse, The Complete Idiot's Guide to Vegan Cooking, The Complete Idiot's Guide to Gluten-Free Vegan Cooking,* and others. She hosts VeganChef.com and lives in Eugene, Oregon.

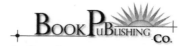

Book Publishing Co.

books that educate, inspire, and empower

All titles in the **Live Healthy Now** series are only **$5.95!**

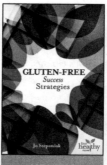

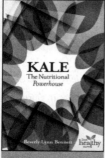

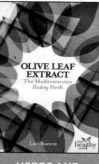

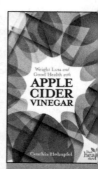

HEALTH ISSUES	HEALTHY FOODS	HERBS AND SUPPLEMENTS	NATURAL SOLUTIONS

A Holistic Approach to **ADHD**

Understanding **GOUT**

WHEAT BELLY Is Modern Wheat Causing Modern Ills?

THE ACID-ALKALINE DIET Balancing the Body Naturally

Enhance Your Health with **FERMENTED FOODS**

GREEN SMOOTHIES The Easy Way to Get Your Greens

PALEO Smoothies

Refreshing Fruit and Vegetable **SMOOTHIES**

AROMATHERAPY Essential Oils for Healing

Healthy and Beautiful with **COCONUT OIL**

The Weekend **DETOX**

Improve Digestion with **FOOD COMBINING**

The Healing Power of **TURMERIC**

Interested in other health topics or healthy cookbooks? See our complete line of titles at **BookPubCo.com** or order directly from:
Book Publishing Company • PO Box 99 • Summertown, TN 38483 • 1-888-260-8458